JAMES OWEN

D1552169

THE

GLUCOSE

MASTER

ACCURATE SUGAR LEVEL

INTRODUCTION

Glucose levels are a fundamental concern for people with diabetes. High glucose, known as hyperglycemia, happens when a specific's glucose is in excess of 180 milligrams for every deciliter. High glucose levels can be unsafe while maybe not quickly guided and lead to both present second and critical length issues. In this article, we see substitute ways to deal with assisting individuals with chopping down their glucose levels. These strategies join the way of life changes, diet tips, and ordinary fixes. Keeping blood sugars at target levels helps people with diabetes avoid certified complexities of contamination. High glucose can cause many cleared-out impacts, which can be unexpected, like horrendous improvement in the circulatory structure, or happen little by a little long haul. Long haul, keeping glucose at unhealthful levels can sting almost nothing and colossal veins in two or three organs and designs, affecting credible results, by keeping glucose levels under 100 mg going before eating and under 180 mg coming after eating, individuals with diabetes can fundamentally diminish their bet of unfriendly impacts from the issue.

☐

☐

CHAPTER ONE

PURPOSES BEHIND HIGH GLUCOSE LEVEL

PANCREATIC DISEASES

Pancreatic afflictions like pancreatitis, pancreatic illness, and cystic fibrosis can cause hyperglycemia since pancreas cells are hurt in these conditions. Insulin is made and liberated from the cells of the pancreas. With irritation and mischief to the pancreas, pancreatic cells are as of now not prepared to convey adequate insulin to kill glucose from the blood to control glucose.

POLYCYSTIC OVARIAN SYNDROME

Polycystic ovary jumble is a condition that causes inconsistent, consistently significant female periods. It is a normal endocrine issue among women of conceptive age. Women with PCOS have hormonal unbalanced attributes, such as extended levels of testosterone, insulin, and combustible proteins called cytokines set liberated from fat tissue. Despite extended levels of insulin, women with PCOS show insulin resistance since their insulin synthetic compounds can't sufficiently take up glucose or use it for energy. Insulin receptors in women with PCOS can't actually bind to insulin. Since insulin transports glucose, a flood of glucose stays in the dispersal system, conveying hyperglycemia.

TRAUMA
Genuine tension in the body, including injury, utilization, and various injuries, can cause high glucose by it is utilized to fundamentally impact how glucose is, stress-induced hyperglycemia results when real stressors to the body enliven

extended development of the smart tactile framework, the body's instinctual response, to convey cytokines and synthetics that actually look at the impacts of insulin in getting rid of flood glucose from the circulatory system. These cytokines and synthetics like epinephrine increase the formation of glucose through the breakdown of glycogen stores into glucose and the change of non-carb sources into glucose. Extended levels of the tension substance cortisol, which is in like manner conveyed, block the effects of insulin from taking glucose from the dissemination framework into cells, further adding to high glucose.

SURGERY AND STRESS

Adjustments to glucose assimilation that occur from genuine strain on the body furthermore occur after an operation. The operation is a controlled sort of tension on the body that results in similar extensions in cytokines and synthetic substances that drive the formation of glucose in the liver and square the effects of insulin by dispensing with the overflow of glucose from the blood. Up to thirty percent of patients can encourage pressure impelled hyperglycemia after an operation, with blood glucose levels that stay brought long up following returning from the facility. Raised glucose after an operation can in a general sense influence all things considered prosperity and constructs the bet of making diabetes and other troublesome conditions.

INFECTIONS
Stress actuated hyperglycemia can moreover result from the real strain of having an infection, similar to pneumonia or urinary parcel defilements. Extended levels of the tension synthetic cortisol that occurs

with infections block the limit of insulin to take out the excess glucose from the circulatory framework, keeping the body in a state of high glucose. High blood glucose in like manner results from infections as a standard reaction to assist the necessities of organs with loving the psyche, kidneys, and red platelets that depend upon glucose for energy to assist the insusceptible design's reaction with deflecting polluting.

MEDICATION SIDE EFFECTS

Certain remedies, for instance, catecholamine vasopressors like dopamine and norepinephrine, immunosuppressants like tacrolimus and cyclosporine, and corticosteroids would addition be able to blood glucose levels by starting synthetic compounds that augmentation blood glucose levels and disturb the conveyance and development of insulin to take up glucose from the blood. Hospitalized patients helping sustenance through an IV may similarly be at an extended bet of making hyperglycemia, as the restorative fluid contains a sugar reply to help with restoring electrolyte balance. The centralization of this fluid should be carefully checked in patients who are debilitated or recovering from an operation or injury to thwart further spikes in glucose.

OBESITY

High glucose is connected with bulkiness since plentiful fat cells upset the agreement between glucose and insulin. An excess of fat cells called adipocytes releases combustible proteins, for instance, interleukins and development decay factor, which increase the body's insurance from insulin by authorizing processes that upset the body's ability to make and convey insulin when glucose is high.

The wealth of fat cells moreover declines the ability to dispense with glucose from the blood to be used for energy or set aside as glycogen inside skeletal muscles. With stoutness, broadened lipids, or unsaturated fat particles, layout pathways that disable insulin motioning inside muscles.

LACK OF PHYSICAL ACTIVITY
The shortfall of dynamic work can grow your glucose, as skeletal muscles are an essential piece of the body that includes glucose for energy or stores extra glucose as glycogen for quite a while later on. With low levels of dynamic work, the muscles become idle and don't take out glucose really from the blood. Standard movement can help with cutting down glucose levels by extending the necessity for muscles to kill glucose from the blood to use for energy.

□

CHAPTER TWO

INCIDENTAL EFFECTS

THIRST

Thirst is the vibe of hoping to drink something. It occurs whenever the body is got dried out regardless. Any condition that can achieve a lack of body water can provoke thirst or pointless thirst. Consequently, thirst is a brand name result of explicit illnesses, most strikingly diabetes mellitus. Thirst is the craving for consumable fluids, achieving the major motivation of animals to drink. It is a central instrument related to fluid balance. It rises up out of a shortfall of fluids or an extension in the gathering of certain osmolites, similar to sodium. If the water volume of the body falls under a particular breaking point or the osmolyte obsession ends up being unreasonably high, structures in the frontal cortex perceive changes in blood constituents and sign thirst. Consistent drying out can cause exceptional and decided afflictions, regardless, which are most frequently connected with renal and neurological issues. Outrageous thirst, called polydipsia, close by ludicrous pee, known as polyuria, may be an indication of diabetes mellitus or diabetes insipid.

SHORTCOMING

Weariness depicts a state of drowsiness that doesn't resolve with rest or rest. Generally speaking use, the shortcoming is indivisible from unbelievable laziness or weakness that ordinarily follows deferred physical or mental development. Right when it doesn't resolve after rest or rest or happens independently of physical or mental exertion, it may be a result of an infirmity that could become outrageous or moderate. Shortcoming can be a part of a mental issue like awfulness may be connected with conditions of consistent misery, for instance, fibromyalgia it could similarly incorporate conditions of progressing low level aggravation, and be an infection related incidental effect in various conditions. Weariness regularly has no alluded to cause and is seen as being outstandingly astounding in nature. Fatigability depicts a shortcoming to exhaustion.

FRUITLESSNESS

Fruitlessness is the disappointment of an individual, animal, or plant to copy by standard means. It is for the most part not the typical state of a strong adult, except for astoundingly among certain eusocial species. It is at any rate the sound state of a human young person or other energetic successors, for they have not yet gone through youthfulness, the body's start of as far as possible. In individuals, desolateness is the frailty to become pregnant following one year of unprotected and standard sex including a male and a female assistant. There are many purposes behind fruitlessness, including some that clinical intercession can treat. Checks suggest that worldwide around five percent of all hetero couples certainly oppose infertility.

SKIN BREAK OUT

Skin breakout, in any case, called skin aggravation Vulgaris, is an excessively long skin condition that happens when dead skin cells and oil from the skin hinder hair follicles. Typical components of the condition consolidate obstructed pores or whiteheads, pimples, smooth skin, and possible scarring. It generally impacts skin with a respectably large number of oil organs, including the face, upper piece of the chest, and back. The resulting appearance can provoke apprehension, diminished certainty, and, in unbelievable cases, misery or contemplations of implosion. Medicines for skin break out are accessible, including way of life changes, prescriptions, and assignments. Eating less fundamental carbs, for instance, sugar could restrict the condition.

CRIMPS

Wrinkle, regardless, called a rhytide, is a get over, edge, or crimp in an all things considered smooth surface, for example, on skin or surface. Skin wrinkles routinely appear considering creating cycles, for example, glycation, reliable resting positions, lack of weight, sun hurt, or quickly, as the result of conceded submersion in water. Age wrinkling in the skin is progressed by steady looks, developing, sun hurt, smoking, awful hydration, and various factors. In individuals, it can moreover be prevented to some degree by avoiding pointless sun based receptiveness and overflow of sugar utilization.

WANTS

A food craving also called specific hunger is a significant yearning to eat up a specific food and isn't exactly equivalent to anticipated hunger. It could be associated with unequivocal desire, the drive to consume explicit enhancements that are a lot of consideration in animals. Food craving is a strong desire to eat a particular sort of food. This need can give off an impression of being wild, and the singular's desire may not be satisfied until they get that particular food. Food assortments with raised levels of sugar glucose, similar to chocolate, are more routinely yearned for than food sources with lower sugar glucose, similar to broccoli, since when glucose interacts with the opiate receptor structure in the psyche a propensity framing setting off sway occurs. The purchaser of the glucose needs to finish more glucose, like a boozer, because the brain has become adjusted to convey happy synthetics each time glucose is accessible.

CHAPTER THREE

THE MOST EFFECTIVE METHOD TO CONTROL GLUCOSE LEVEL

SCREEN GLUCOSE LEVELS INTENTLY

High glucose levels regularly don't cause accidental impacts until they run far more than 200 mg. At that breaking point, it is head for an individual with diabetes to screen their glucose two or multiple times consistently. Doing such won't propose that glucose levels anytime get that high. A person with diabetes can use a home glucose screen to check glucose levels. Considerations for how ceaselessly to check glucose levels during the day will vacillate starting with one individual and afterward onto the accompanying. A specialist can make the best suggestions concerning glucose checking for an individual with diabetes.

DECLINE SUGAR ADMISSION

Eating a low-carb, high-protein diet decreases glucose levels. The body limits carbs into sugar that the body uses as energy. Some carbs are huge in the eating plan. Notwithstanding, for individuals with diabetes, eating a superfluous number of carbs can make glucose spikes nonsensically high. Reducing the extents of carbs a solitary eats diminishes how much a particular's glucose spikes.

EAT THE RIGHT SUGARS

Direct starches are generally included one sort of sugar. They are found in food sources, like white bread, pasta, and candy. The body separates these starches into sugar quickly, which causes glucose levels to rapidly rise. Complex carbs are incorporated something like three sugars that are related together. Since the planned eminence care aftereffects of such starches are perplexed, it takes the body longer to separate them. Appropriately, sugar is conveyed into the body considerably more little by little, proposing that glucose levels don't quickly climb following eating them. Instances of tangled starches join entire grain oats and yams.

KEEP A SOUND WEIGHT

Acquiring thin aides impacts glucose levels. Being overweight is connected with widened episodes of diabetes and more fundamental occasions of insulin resistance. It is basic to see that an individual doesn't need to achieve ideal body weight to benefit from shedding 10 to 20 pounds and keeping it off. Doing such will in a like way further cultivate cholesterol, decline the bet of intricacies, and work on a solitary's overall vibe of thriving. Eating a vitalizing eating routine spilling over with verdant food assortments and getting sufficient development can assist an individual with shedding pounds or remaining mindful of their right presently sound weight.

CONTROL SEGMENT SIZE

At most meals, an individual ought to see section rules given by a prepared proficient or nutritionist. Glutting at a sitting can cause a spike in glucose. In any case, direct carbs are generally connected with raised glucose levels, all food causes glucose levels to rise. Mindful control of parts can keep glucose levels more controlled.

WORK OUT ROUTINELY

The preparation appreciates many advantages for individuals with diabetes, including weight decline and expanded insulin responsiveness. Insulin is a substance that helps people with withdrawing sugar from the body. People with diabetes either don't make enough or any insulin in their body or are impenetrable to the insulin the body produces. Practice additionally assists with chopping down glucose levels by empowering the body's muscles to incorporate sugar for energy.

HYDRATE

Reasonable hydration is essential to a fortifying way of life. For individuals stressed over chopping down high glucose, it is fundamental. Drinking satisfactory water forestalls drying out and additionally assists the kidneys with taking out added sugar from the body in the pee. Those hoping to lessen glucose levels should seek after water and keep away from every sweet beverage, for example, normal things crushed or pop, which could raise glucose levels considering everything. People with diabetes should diminish alcohol admission to what definitively could analyze one award reliably for women and two for men other than if various impediments apply.

ENDEAVOR HOMEGROWN SEPARATES
Neighborhood improvements, like green tea, may assist with supporting the eating routine with significant upgrades. Neighborhood concentrates could earnestly impact treating and controlling glucose levels. By a wide margin, most should attempt to get upgrades from the food varieties they eat. In any case, supplements are regularly useful for individuals who don't get enough of the improvements from normal sources. Most experts don't consider supplements a treatment without assistance from another person. An individual ought to sort out their focal thought master going preceding taking any redesign, as they

could upset any recommended courses of action.

ADMINISTER PRESSURE

Stress impacts glucose levels. The body exudes tension on engineered substances when under strain, and these manufactured mixtures raise glucose levels. Arranging strain through reflection and exercise can correspondingly assist with slicing down glucose levels.

GET SUFFICIENT REST

Rest assists an individual with decreasing how much sugar is in their blood. Getting satisfactory rest reliably is a mind-boggling procedure for assisting keep with blooding sugar levels at a typical level. Glucose levels will all over flood in the early morning hours. In a great number of individuals, insulin will show the body glucose, which keeps the glucose levels conventional. The setback of rest can almost influence insulin obstruction, recommending that a particular's glucose level could spike essentially from the deficiency of rest.

☐

CHAPTER FOUR

DIET FOR BLOOD SUGAR LEVEL

FISH

Fish, including fish and shellfish, offer a critical wellspring of protein, sound fats, supplements, minerals, and disease avoidance specialists that could help with coordinating glucose levels. Protein is the principal for glucose control. It moves back digestion and thwarts post-feast glucose spikes, as well as extends impressions of entirety. Additionally, it could help with hindering pigging out and propelling excess muscle versus fat incident, two effects that are major for strong glucose levels. A high affirmation of oily fish like salmon and sardines has been shown to help with additional creating glucose rules.

PUMPKIN AND PUMPKIN SEEDS

Greatly hidden and stacked with fiber and infection expectation subject matter experts, pumpkin is an incomprehensible decision for glucose rule. All things considered, pumpkin is utilized as a standard diabetic fix in different nations like Mexico and Iran. Pumpkin is high in carbs called polysaccharides, which have been perused up for their glucose coordinating potential. Drugs with pumpkin focuses and powders have been shown to in a general sense decrease glucose levels in both human and animal investigations. Notwithstanding, more examination should finish up how the entire pumpkin, like when it's eaten cooked or steamed, may help glucose. Pumpkin seeds are stacked with strong fats and proteins, seeking after them a brilliant choice for glucose control as well.

NUTS AND NUT MARGARINE

Research has shown that eating nuts may be a convincing technique for controlling glucose levels. An audit of twenty-five people with type2 diabetes showed that consuming the two peanuts and almonds throughout the span of the day as an element of a low-carb diet diminished both fasting and post-feast glucose levels.

OKRA

Okra is a characteristic item that is generally utilized as a vegetable. It's a rich wellspring of glucose cutting down strengthens like polysaccharides and flavonoid disease counteraction specialists. In Turkey, okra seeds have for quite a while been used as a trademark answer for treating diabetes in view of their solid glucose cutting down properties. Rhamnogalacturonan, the main polysaccharide in okra, has been recognized as a solid enemy of diabetic compounds. Okra contains the flavonoids isoquercitrin and quercetin which help with decreasing glucose by controlling explicit mixtures.

FLAXSEEDS

Flax seeds are affluent in fiber and strong fats and outstanding for their clinical benefits. Specifically, flax seeds could help with lessening glucose levels. In an 8 week study in 57 people with type2 diabetes, individuals who consumes fat yogurt containing 30 grams of flax seeds every day experienced colossal declines in HbA1c, differentiated and individuals who consumed plain yogurt. Moreover, an overview of 25 controlled examinations found that eating whole flax seeds incited basic upgrades in glucose control.

BEANS AND LENTILS

Beans and lentils are rich in supplements, similar to magnesium, fiber, and protein, that can help with cutting down glucose. They're particularly high in dissolvable fiber and safe starch, which help with moving back absorption and may additionally foster glucose response after suppers. For example, an audit of 12 women showed that adding dim beans or chickpeas to a rice supper by and large diminished post-dinner glucose levels, differentiated and eating rice alone. Various assessments have shown that eating beans and lentils wouldn't simply advantage having the option to glucose rules yet moreover possibly help protect against the headway of diabetes.

AVOCADOS

As well as being rich and great, avocados could offer basic benefits for glucose rules. They're adequate in solid fats, fiber, enhancements, and minerals, and adding them to dinners has been displayed to furthermore encourage glucose levels. Different assessments have seen that avocados could help with diminishing glucose levels and shield against the improvement of metabolic issue, which is a lot of conditions, including hypertension and high glucose, that increases progressing contamination risk. Regardless, recall that numerous assessments that have investigated the effects of avocado confirmation on glucose levels were funded by the Hass Avocado Board, which could have impacted pieces of the examinations.

OATS AND OAT WHEAT

Recalling oats and oat wheat for your eating routine could help with additional fostering your glucose levels in light of their high joy of dissolvable fiber, which has been shown to have enormous glucose diminishing properties. An assessment of 16 examinations found that oat confirmation basically diminished HbA1c and fasting glucose levels, differentiated and controlled dinners.

CONCLUSION

High glucose can result from an assortment of causes, not simply diabetes. You don't have to live with diabetes to cultivate hyperglycemia. Having high glucose can assemble your bet of making diabetes and related intricacies later on. A mix of elements can add to high glucose, and some of them like eating routine and exercise can assist with holding your blood glucose in line. Now and again high glucose in people without diabetes could be anticipated as pre-diabetes, which could provoke the improvement of diabetes.

Expecting you have high glucose routinely, it's crucial to check with your clinical benefits provider and screen it. Diet accepts a basic part in the improvement of high glucose. Excess usage of sugar and carb-containing food sources brings glucose steps up directly following eating as the food is isolated into glucose particles that enter the course framework. In a sound individual, the presence of more glucose particles in the blood signals the pancreas to convey insulin, which helps take up glucose from the blood and transports it to the muscles and liver to be used for energy and limit. As glucose reduces, the signs to the pancreas to convey more insulin stop, and glucose levels should return to a consistent benchmark. At the point when levels of glucose reliably become raised with repeat and ludicrous sugar and carb use, the wealth of glucose in the course framework vitalizes the pancreas to convey a huge load of insulin. For a really long time, the body stops noting insulin due to determining high glucose, causing insulin obstacles, and keeping glucose high. Managing a strong and offset diet with proteins, fats, and fiber-rich food sources while confining sugar and taking care of refined starches can help with controlling glucose levels. Abundance liquor utilization can additionally affect your glucose by preventing your liver's capacity to manage the creation and presence of glucose and inimically impact your body's reaction to insulin.

Made in the USA
Coppell, TX
01 May 2022

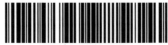

77298370R00024